The Complete Gu

Cooking

Tasty and Easy Recipes to Discover New Meals and
Boost Your Appetite

Tim Singhapat

Table of contents

BARBECUED PORK ON RICE

Ingredients:

- 1 cucumber, thinly cut
- 1 green onion, trimmed and thinly cut
- 1 hard-boiled egg, peeled
- 1 pork tenderloin, trimmed of surplus fat
- 1 tablespoon sesame seeds, toasted
- 1 teaspoon Chinese 5-spice powder
- 1½ cups water
- 2 tablespoons flour
- 2 tablespoons rice vinegar
- 2 tablespoons soy sauce
- 2 tablespoons sugar
  Jasmine rice, cooked in accordance with
- package directions

Directions:

1. Cut the tenderloin into medallions roughly ¼-inch thick. Put the medallions in a mixing container.
2. Mix the sugar, soy sauce, and 5-spice powder in a small container.
3. Pour the soy mixture over pork strips and toss the strips until meticulously coated. Let marinate minimum 30 minutes, but if possible overnight.
4. Preheat your oven to 350 degrees. Put the pork pieces in a single layer on a baking sheet lined using foil. Reserve any remaining marinade.
5. Bake the pork for roughly 1 hour. The pork with be firm and rather dry, but

not burned. It will also have a reddish color.

6. Put the reserved marinade in a small deep cooking pan and heat to boiling. Remove the heat and put in the peeled egg, rolling it in the sauce to color it. Take away the egg and set it aside. When sufficiently cool to handle, cut it into thin pieces.

7. Mix the flour and water, and put in it to the marinade. Bring to its boiling point to thicken, then turn off the heat.

8. Put in the vinegar and the sesame seeds. Adjust seasoning by putting in additional sugar and/or soy sauce.

9. To serve, place some Jasmine rice in the middle of each plate. Fan a few pieces of the pork around 1 side of the rice. Fan some cucumber slices and cut hard-boiled egg around the other side.

   Ladle some of the sauce over the pork and drizzle with the green onion slices.

Yield: Servings 2–3

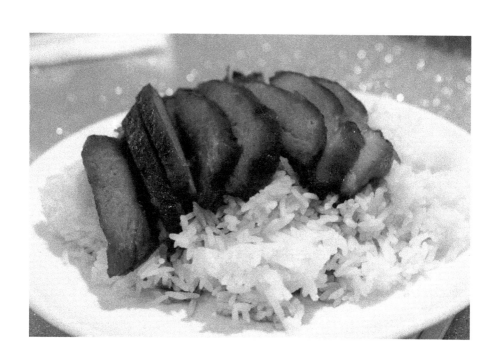

LEMONGRASS PORK

Ingredients:

- ¼ cup chopped shallots
- ¼ cup coconut milk
- ¼ cup minced garlic
- ¼ cup whiskey
- ½ cup brown sugar
- ½ cup chopped lemongrass stalks (inner white portion only)
- ½ cup dark soy sauce
- ½ cup fish sauce
- 1 pound lean pork, cut into bite-sized pieces
- 1 teaspoon cayenne pepper
- 3 tablespoons sesame oil

Directions:

1. In a moderate-sized-sized deep cooking pan, mix the brown sugar, fish sauce, soy sauce, lemongrass, whiskey, shallots, and garlic. Over moderate heat, bring to its boiling point and cook until the mixture is reduced to half. Take away the marinade from the heat and let it cool to room temperature. Mix in the coconut milk, sesame oil, and cayenne pepper.
2. Put the pork and the marinade in a big Ziplock bag. Marinate the pork in your fridge for minimum three hours, or overnight.
3. Drain the meat, saving for later the marinade. Thread the meat onto metal skewers (or soaked bamboo skewers), and grill or broil to your preference.

4. Put the reserved marinade in a small deep cooking pan and bring it to its boiling point on moderate to high heat. Lower the heat and simmer the marinade for two to three minutes. Use the marinade as a dipping sauce for the pork.

Yield: Servings 2

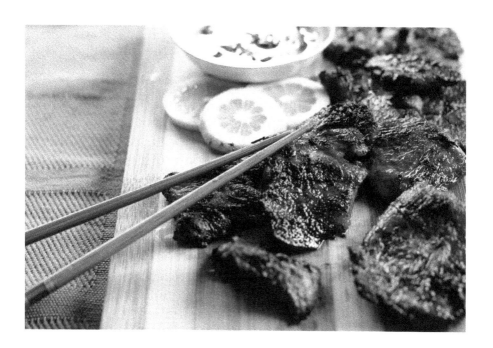

PORK AND SPINACH CURRY

Ingredients:

- ½ cup lean pork strips
- ½ lime
- ½ pound baby spinach
- 1 cup coconut milk, divided
- 1 tablespoon Red Curry Paste (Page 17)
- 2 cups water
- 2 tablespoons sugar
- 3–4 kaffir lime leaves, crumbled
- 4 tablespoons fish sauce
  Rice, cooked in accordance with package
- directions

Directions:

1. In a moderate-sized-sized deep cooking pan, heat ½ cup of the coconut milk and the curry paste on moderate to low heat, stirring to blend meticulously. Cook for five minutes, stirring continuously, so that the sauce does not burn.
2. Put in the pork cubes, the rest of the coconut milk, and the water. Return the mixture to a simmer and allow to cook for five minutes. Squeeze the juice of the lime half into the curry. Put in the lime half.
3. Mix in the kaffir lime leaves, fish sauce, and sugar. Continue simmering for five to 10 more minutes or until the pork is thoroughly cooked. Take away the lime half.

Yield: Servings 1–2

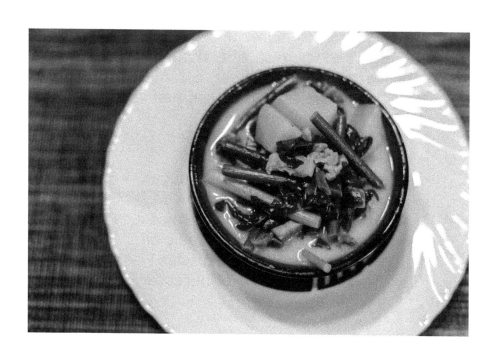

THAI-STYLE BEEF WITH BROCCOLI

Ingredients:

- ½ of a 7–8-ounce package of rice sticks 1 cup broccoli pieces
- 1 medium shallot, chopped
- 1 pound lean beef, cut into bite-sized pieces
- 1 tablespoon preserved soy beans (not necessary)
- 1 teaspoon chili powder
- 2 cups water
- 2 tablespoons brown sugar
- 2 tablespoons fish sauce
- 2 tablespoons sweet soy sauce
- 3 tablespoons vegetable oil
- Hot sauce (not necessary)
- Lime wedges (not necessary)

Directions:

1. Heat the vegetable oil in a wok on moderate to high heat. Put in the shallot and stir-fry until it starts to become tender. Put in the chili powder and continue to stir-fry until well blended.

2. Put in the brown sugar, fish sauce, soy sauce, and soy beans; stir-fry for half a minute.
3. Put in the beef and continue to stir-fry until the beef is almost done, roughly two minutes.
4. Mix in the water and bring it to its boiling point. Put in the rice sticks, stirring until they start to cook. Lower the heat to moderate, cover, and allow to cook for half a minute. Stir and decrease the heat to moderate-low, cover, and allow to cook for about three minutes.
5. Put in the broccoli pieces, cover, and cook for a minute. Take
away the wok from the heat and tweak seasoning to taste.
6. Serve with wedges of lime and hot sauce passed separately at the table.

Yield: Servings 2–4

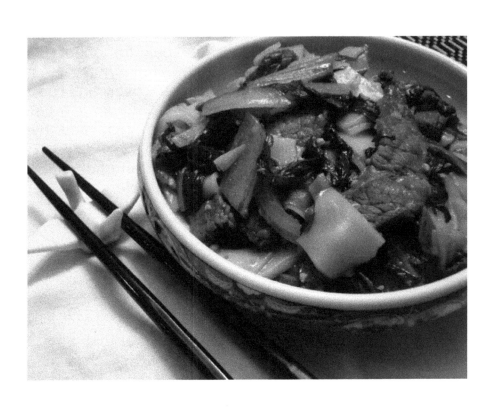

PORK WITH TOMATOES AND STICKY RICE

Ingredients:

- ½ pound crudely chopped lean pork
- ½ teaspoon salt
- ½ teaspoon shrimp paste
- 1 tablespoon chopped garlic
- 1 tablespoon fish sauce
- 1 tablespoon vegetable oil
- 1 teaspoon brown sugar
- 2 tablespoons chopped shallot
- 20 cherry tomatoes, quartered
- 7 small dried chilies
- Sticky rice, cooked in accordance with package directions

Directions:

1. Trim the chilies of their stems and shake out the seeds. Cut them into little pieces, cover them with warm water, and allow them to soak for about twenty minutes to tenderize; drain.
2. Using a food processor or mortar and pestle, grind (or process) the chilies and salt together until a thick paste is formed.

Put in the shrimp paste, shallot, and garlic. Process until well blended; set aside.

3. Heat a wok or heavy-bottomed frying pan using low heat. Put in the vegetable oil and heat for a minute. Put in the chili purée and cook for roughly three minutes or until the color of the paste deepens.

4. Raise the heat to moderate and put in the pork; stir-fry for a minute. Put in the tomatoes and carry on cooking for three to four minutes, stirring regularly.

5. Mix in the fish sauce and brown sugar; simmer for a couple of minutes. Adjust seasoning to taste.

6. Serve this beef dish with sticky rice either warm or at room temperature.

Yield: Servings 2

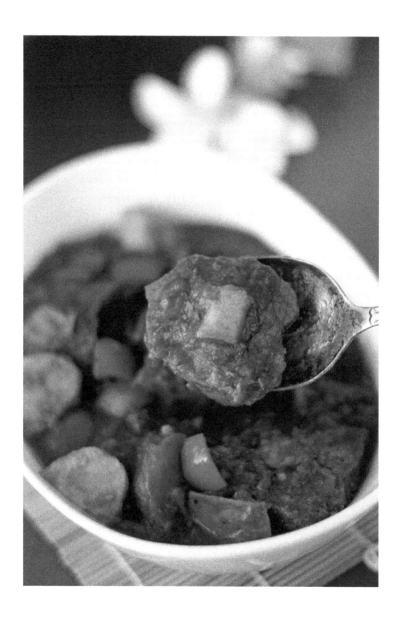

CINNAMON STEWED BEEF

Ingredients:

- 1 (2-inch) piece of cinnamon stick
- 1 bay leaf
- 1 celery stalk, cut
- 1 clove garlic, smashed
- 1 pound beef sirloin, trimmed of all fat and slice into 1-inch cubes
- 1½ quarts water
- 2 tablespoons sugar
- 2 tablespoons sweet soy sauce
- 2 whole star anise
- 5 sprigs cilantro
- 5 tablespoons soy sauce

Directions:

1. Put the water in a big soup pot and bring to its boiling point. Decrease the heat to low and put in the rest of the ingredients.
2. Simmer, putting in more water if required, for minimum 2 hours or until the beef is completely soft. If possible, let the stewed beef sit in your fridge overnight.
3. To serve, place noodles or rice on the bottom of 4 soup bowls. Put in pieces of beef and then ladle broth over. Drizzle with chopped cilantro or cut green onions if you prefer. Pass a vinegar-chili sauce of your choice as a dip for the beef.

Yield: Servings

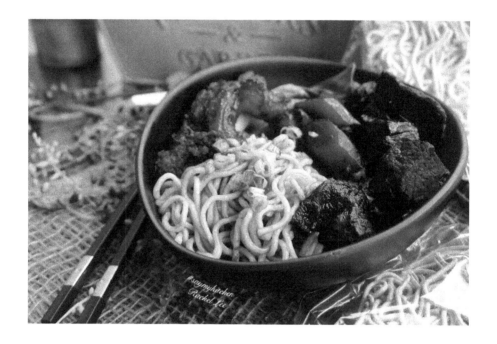

BASIL CHICKEN

Ingredients:

- 1 big onion, cut into thin slices
- 1 tablespoon water
- 1½ cups chopped basil leaves, divided
- 1½ tablespoons soy sauce
- 1½ teaspoons sugar
- 2 tablespoons fish sauce
- 2 tablespoons vegetable oil
- 2 whole boneless, skinless chicken breasts, cut into 1-inch cubes
- 3 cloves garlic, minced
- 3 Thai chilies, seeded and thinly cut

Directions:

1. In a moderate-sized-sized container, mix the fish sauce, the soy sauce, water, and sugar. Put in the chicken cubes and stir to coat. Let marinate for about ten minutes.
2. In a big frying pan or wok, heat oil on moderate to high heat. Put in the onion and stir-fry for two to three minutes. Put in the

chilies and garlic and carry on cooking for another half a minute.
3. Using a slotted spoon, remove the chicken from the marinade and put in it to the frying pan (reserve the marinade.) Stir-fry until almost thoroughly cooked, approximately 3 minutes.
4. Put in the reserved marinade and cook for another half a minute. Take away the frying pan from the heat and mix in 1 cup of the basil.
5. Decorate using the rest of the basil, and serve with rice.

Yield: Servings 4

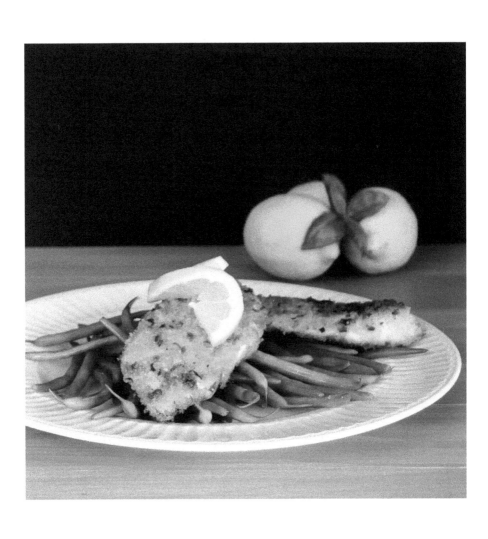

BRANDIED CHICKEN

Ingredients:

- ¼ cup vegetable oil
- 1 (1-inch) piece ginger, cut
- 1 teaspoon salt
- 1 whole roasting chicken, washed and trimmed of surplus fat
- 2 shots brandy
- 2 tablespoons black soy sauce
- 6 tablespoons soy sauce
- 8 cloves garlic, minced

Directions:

1. Fill a pot big enough to hold the whole chicken roughly full of water. Bring the water to its boiling point using high heat. Lower the heat to moderate and cautiously put in the chicken to the pot. Regulate the heat so that the water is just simmering.

2. Poach the whole chicken for twenty minutes to half an hour or until thoroughly cooked. Cautiously remove the chicken from the pot, ensuring to drain the hot water from the cavity of the bird. Position the chicken aside to cool.
3. Take away the skin from the bird and discard. Take away the meat from the chicken and cut it into 1-inch pieces; set aside. (This portion of the recipe can be done 1 or 2 days in advance.)
4. Put in the oil to a big frying pan or wok and heat on medium. Put in the soy sauces, salt, and garlic. Stir-fry until the garlic starts to tenderize, approximately half a minute to one minute.
5. Put in the chicken pieces, stirring to coat. Mix in the brandy and the ginger.
6. Cover the frying pan or wok, decrease the heat to low, and simmer five to ten more minutes.

Yield: Servings 4–6

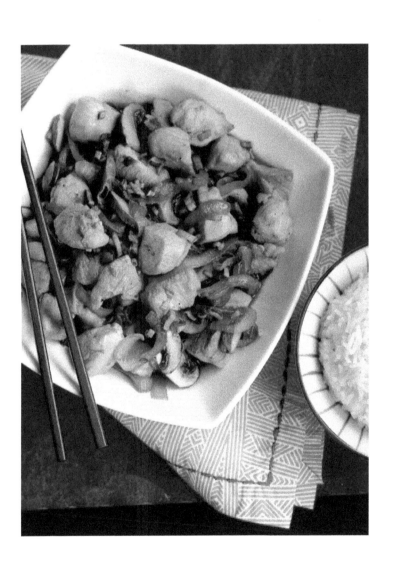

CHICKEN WITH BLACK PEPPER AND GARLIC

Ingredients:

- 1 cup fish sauce
- 1 tablespoon whole black peppercorns
- 1 teaspoon sugar
- 2 pounds boneless, skinless chicken breasts, cut into strips
- 3 tablespoons vegetable oil
- 5 cloves garlic, cut in half

Directions:

1. Using either a mortar and pestle or a food processor, mix the black peppercorns with the garlic.
2. Put the chicken strips in a big mixing container. Put in the garlic-pepper mixture and the fish sauce, and stir until blended.
3. Cover the container, place in your fridge, and let marinate for twenty minutes to half an hour.
4. Heat the vegetable oil on moderate heat in a wok or frying pan. When it is hot, put in the chicken mixture and stir-fry until thoroughly cooked, approximately 3 to five minutes.
5. Mix in the sugar. Put in additional sugar or fish sauce to taste.

Yield: Servings 4–6

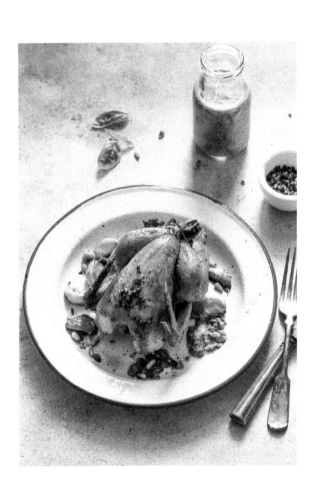

CHILI-FRIED CHICKEN

Ingredients:

- ½ teaspoon ground coriander
- ½ teaspoon white pepper
- 1½ teaspoons salt, divided
- 2 small onions, thinly cut
- 2 tablespoons vegetable oil
  3 pounds chicken pieces, washed and patted dry 3 tablespoons <u>Tamarind Concentrate</u>
- <u>(Page 20)</u>
- 8 big red chilies, seeded and chopped
- Pinch of turmeric
- Vegetable oil for deep-frying

Directions:

1. In a small container mix the tamarind, turmeric, coriander, 1 teaspoon of the salt, and the pepper.
2. Put the chicken pieces in a big Ziplock bag. Pour the tamarind mixture over the chicken, seal the bag, and marinate minimum 2 hours or overnight in your fridge.
3. In a small sauté pan, heat 2 tablespoons of vegetable oil on moderate heat. Put in the red chilies, onions, and the rest of the salt;

sauté for five minutes. Set aside to cool slightly.
4. Move the chili mixture to a food processor and pulse for a short period of time to make a coarse sauce.
5. Drain the chicken and discard the marinade. Deep-fry the chicken pieces in hot oil until the skin is golden and the bones are crunchy. Take away the cooked chicken to paper towels to drain.
6. Put the cooked chicken in a big mixing container. Pour the chili sauce over the chicken and toss until each piece is uniformly coated.

Yield: Servings 4–6

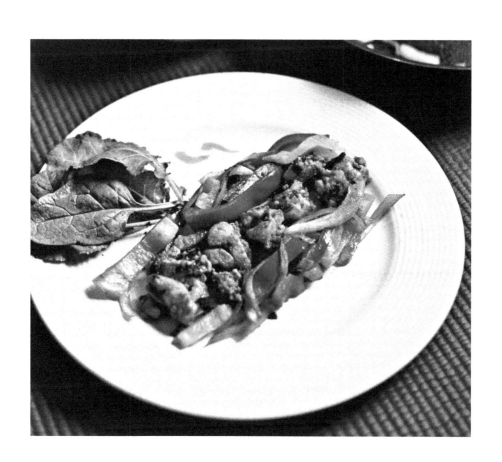

FRAGRANT ROAST CHICKEN

Ingredients:

For the marinade:

- ½ cup fish sauce
- ½ cup sweet dark soy sauce
- 1 tablespoon freshly ground black pepper
- 2 tablespoons crushed garlic
- 2 tablespoons freshly grated gingerroot

For the stuffing:

- ½ cup chopped cilantro
- ½ cup chopped mushrooms
- ½ cup cut bruised lemongrass stalks
- ½ cup fresh grated galangal
- ½ cup freshly grated ginger
- 1 roasting chicken, cleaned and patted dry

Directions:

1. Mix all of the marinade ingredients in a plastic bag big enough to hold the whole chicken. Put in the chicken, ensuring to coat the whole bird with the marinade. Put the chicken in your fridge and leave overnight.
2. Take away the chicken from the plastic bag, saving for later the marinade.
3. Put all of the stuffing ingredients in a big mixing container. Mix in the reserved marinade.
4. Fill the bird's cavity and place it breast side up in a roasting pan. Put the roasting pan in a preheated 400 degree oven and roast for 50 to 60 minutes, or until the juices run clear.

Yield: Servings 2–4

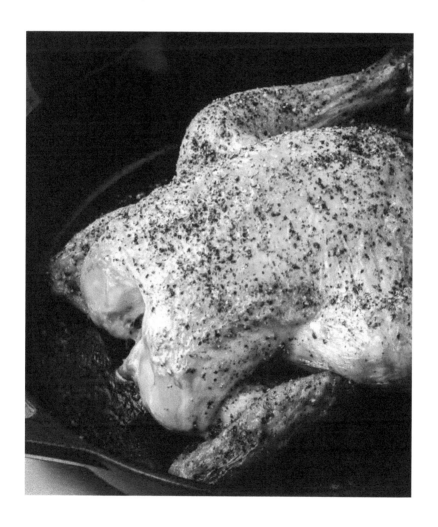

GINGER CHICKEN

Ingredients:

- 1 cup cut domestic mushrooms
- 1 tablespoon chopped garlic
- 1 whole boneless, skinless chicken breast, cut into bite-sized pieces
- 2 tablespoons dark soy sauce
- 2 tablespoons fish sauce
- 2 tablespoons oyster sauce
- 2–3 habanero or bird's eye chilis
- 3 green onions, trimmed and slice into 1-inch pieces
- 3 tablespoons chopped onion
- 3 tablespoons grated ginger
- 3 tablespoons vegetable oil
- Cilantro
- Jasmine rice, cooked in accordance with package directions Pinch of sugar

Directions:

1. In a small container mix the fish, soy, and oyster sauces; set aside.
2. Heat the oil in a big wok until super hot. Put in the garlic and chicken, and stir-fry just until the chicken starts to change color.
3. Put in the reserved sauce and cook until it starts to simmer while stirring continuously.
4. Put in the mushrooms, ginger, sugar, onion, and chilies; simmer until the chicken is thoroughly cooked, approximately eight minutes.

5. To serve, ladle the chicken over Jasmine rice and top with green onion and cilantro.

Yield: Servings 2

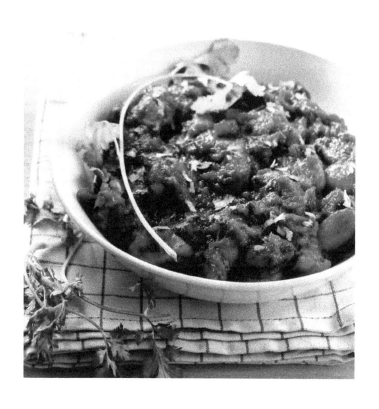

JUNGLE CHICKEN

Ingredients:

- ½ cup coconut milk
- 1 stalk lemongrass, inner portion roughly chopped
- 1 whole boneless, skinless chicken breast, cut into fine strips 10–fifteen
- basil leaves
- 2 (2-inch-long, ½-inch wide) strips of lime peel
- 2 tablespoons vegetable oil
- 2–4 serrano chilies, stems and seeds removed 2–4 tablespoons

Directions:

1. Put the chilies, lemongrass, and lime peel into a food processor and pulse until ground.
2. Heat the oil on moderate to high heat in a wok or big frying pan. Put in the chili mixture and sauté for one to two minutes.
3. Mix in the coconut milk and cook for a couple of minutes.
4. Put in the chicken and cook until the chicken is thoroughly cooked, approximately five minutes.
5. Decrease the heat to low and put in the fish sauce and basil leaves to taste.
6. Serve with sufficient Jasmine rice.

Yield: Servings 2–3

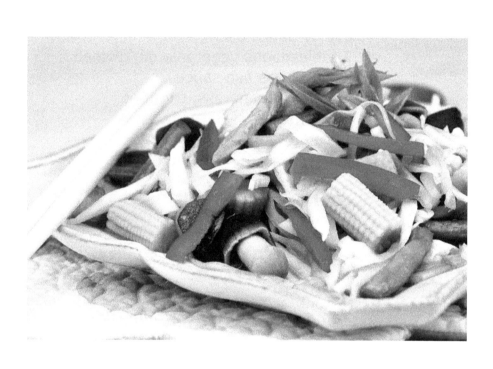

LEMONGRASS CHICKEN SKEWERS

Ingredients:

- 12 big cubes chicken breast meat, a little over 1 ounce each
- 2 tablespoons vegetable oil, divided
- 2 teaspoons fish sauce
- 5 stalks lemongrass, trimmed
- Black pepper
- Juice of 1 lime
- Pinch of dried red pepper flakes
- Pinch of sugar
- Sea salt to taste

Directions:

1. Remove 2 inches from the thick end of each stalk of lemongrass; set aside. Bruise 4 of the lemongrass stalks using the back of a knife. Take away the tough outer layer of the fifth stalk, exposing the soft core; mince.
2. Skewer 3 cubes of chicken on each lemongrass stalk. Drizzle the skewers with the minced lemongrass and black pepper, and sprinkle with 1 tablespoon of oil. Cover using plastic wrap and place in your fridge for twelve to one day.
3. Chop all of the reserved lemongrass stalk ends. Put in a small deep cooking pan and cover with water. Bring to its boiling point,

cover, and let reduce until roughly 2 tablespoons of liquid is left; strain. Return the liquid to the deep cooking pan and further reduce to 1 tablespoon.

4. Mix the lemongrass liquid with the red pepper flakes, lime juice, fish sauce, sugar, and remaining tablespoon of oil; set aside.
5. Prepare a grill to high heat. Grill the chicken skewers for roughly two to three minutes per side, or until done to your preference.
6. To serve, spoon a little of the lemongrass sauce over the top of each skewer and drizzle with sea salt.

Yield: Servings 4

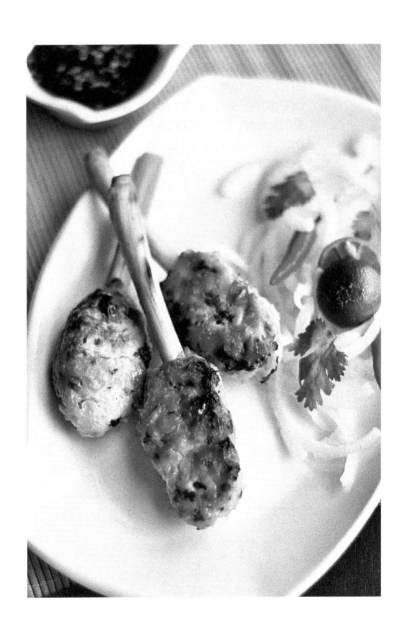

RED CHILI CHICKEN

Ingredients:

- 1 tablespoon vegetable oil
- ½ cup coconut milk
- 1 whole boneless, skinless chicken breast, cut into bite-sized pieces
- 2 kaffir lime leaves or 2 (2-inch-long, ½-inch wide) pieces of lime zest
- 1 tablespoon basil leaves
- 2 tablespoons fish sauce
- 1 tablespoon brown sugar
- 4 ounces Thai eggplant (green peas can be substituted)
- 1–3 tablespoons Red Curry Paste (Page 17)

Directions:

1. In a big frying pan or wok, heat the oil on moderate to high heat. Mix in the curry paste and cook until aromatic, approximately one minute.

2. Lower the heat to moderate-low and put in the coconut milk. Stirring continuously, cook until a thin film of oil develops on the surface.
3. Put in all of the rest of the ingredients except the eggplant. Bring to its boiling point, reduce heat, and simmer until the chicken starts to turn opaque, approximately five minutes.
4. Put in the eggplant and carry on cooking until the chicken is done to your preference, approximately 3 minutes more.

Yield: Servings 2

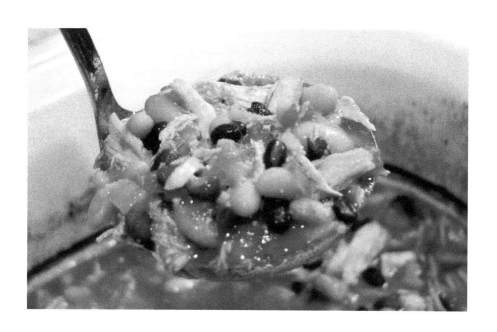

SIAMESE ROAST CHICKEN

Ingredients:

- 1 clove garlic, minced
- 1 medium onion, chopped
- 1 tablespoon fish sauce
- 1 teaspoon (or to taste) dried red pepper flakes
- 1 whole roasting chicken
- 2 stalks lemongrass, thinly cut (soft inner core only)
- Salt and pepper to taste
- Vegetable oil

Directions:

1. To prepare the marinade, put the lemongrass, onion, garlic, red pepper, and fish sauce in a food processor. Process until a thick paste is formed. Place in your fridge for minimum 30 minutes, overnight if possible.

2. Spread the marinade throughout the chicken cavity and then drizzle the cavity with salt and pepper. Rub the outside of the bird with a small amount of vegetable oil (or butter if you prefer) and sprinkle with salt and pepper. Put the bird in a roasting pan, and cover it using plastic wrap. Place in your fridge for a few hours to marinate, if possible. Take away the chicken from the fridge roughly thirty minutes before roasting.
3. Preheat your oven to 500 degrees. Take away the plastic wrap and put the bird in your oven, legs first, and roast for 50 to 60 minutes or until the juices run clear.

Yield: Servings 2–4

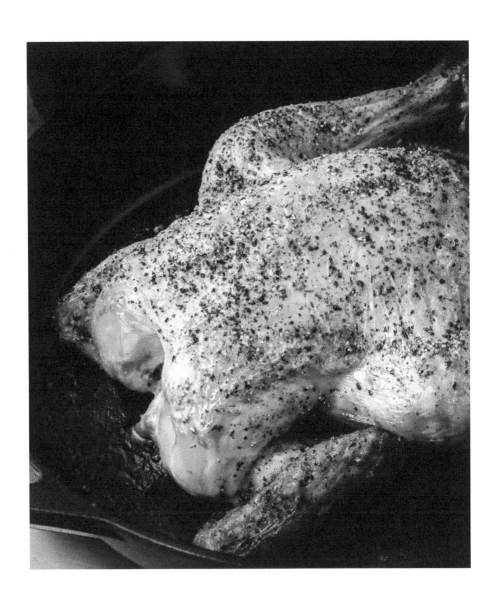

SWEET-AND-SOUR CHICKEN

Ingredients:

- 1 (1-inch) piece of ginger, peeled and minced
- 1 green and 1 red bell pepper, seeded and slice into 1-inch pieces
- 1 pound boneless, skinless chicken breasts, cut into 1-inch cubes
- 1 small onion, thinly cut
- 1 tablespoon vegetable oil
- 1–2 tablespoons prepared chili sauce
- 2 cloves garlic, minced
- 2 tablespoons soy sauce
- 4–6 tablespoons prepared <u>Plum Sauce </u>(Page 34)
- 8 ounces canned pineapple pieces, drained
- Jasmine rice, cooked in accordance with package directions

Directions:

1. In a small container, mix the soy sauce, garlic, ginger, and chili sauce. Put in the chicken pieces, stirring to coat. Set aside to marinate for minimum twenty minutes.
2. Heat the oil in a wok or big frying pan on moderate heat. Put in the onion and sauté until translucent, approximately 3 minutes.
3. Put in the chicken mixture and carry on cooking for another three to five minutes.
4. Put in the bell peppers, the pineapple, and plum sauce. Cook for another five minutes or until the chicken is thoroughly cooked.

5. Serve over lots of fluffy Jasmine rice.

Yield: Servings 4

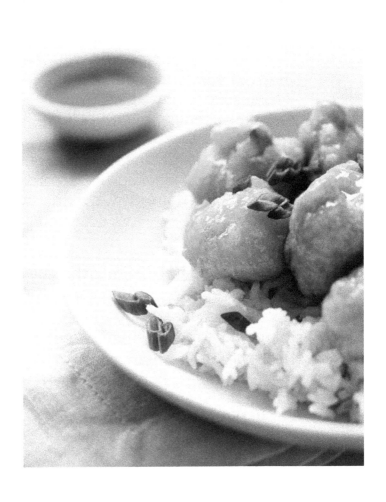

TAMARIND STIR-FRIED CHICKEN WITH MUSHROOMS

Ingredients:

- 2 tablespoons vegetable oil
- Salt and freshly ground black pepper
- 1 teaspoon sugar
- 4 ounces domestic mushrooms, cut
- ½ cup cut onions
- 1 clove garlic, minced
- 2 tablespoons <u>Tamarind Concentrate (Page 20)</u>
- 2 tablespoons water
- 1 cup bean sprouts
- 1 small jalapeño, seeded and minced
- ¼ cup chopped basil
- 1–2 whole boneless, skinless chicken breasts, cut into bite-sized cubes

Directions:

1. Heat the vegetable oil in a big sauté pan or wok using high heat. Flavour the chicken with the salt, pepper, and sugar.
2. Put in the chicken to the pan and stir-fry for a couple of minutes. Put in the mushrooms, onions, and garlic; carry on cooking for another two to three minutes. Put in the tamarind and water; stir.
3. Put in the rest of the ingredients. Adjust seasonings to taste before you serve.

Yield: Servings 1–2

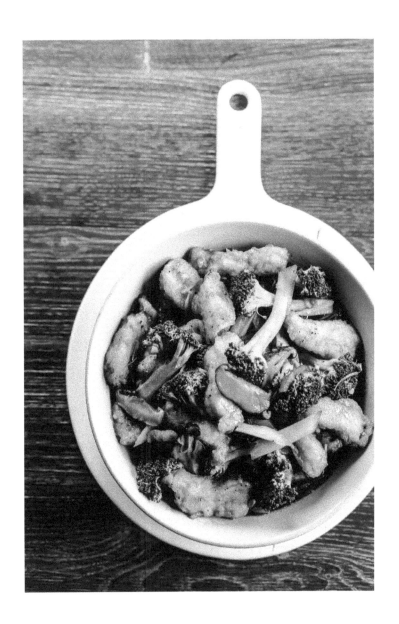

THAI CASHEW CHICKEN

Ingredients:

- 3 tablespoons vegetable oil
- 1 big whole boneless, skinless chicken breast, cut into fine strips
- 4 green onions, trimmed and slice into 1-inch lengths
- 1 small onion, thinly cut
- ¼ cup chicken broth
- 1 tablespoon oyster sauce
- 1 tablespoon fish sauce
- 2 tablespoons sugar
- ¾ cup whole cashews
- 2–3 teaspoons Chili Tamarind Paste (page 11)
- 5–10 dried Thai chilies
- 5–10 cloves garlic, mashed

Directions:

1. In a wok or big frying pan, heat the oil on moderate to high heat until hot.
2. Put in the chilies and stir-fry for a short period of time until they darken in color. Move the chilies to a paper towel to drain; set aside.

3. Put in the garlic to the wok and stir-fry until just starting to turn golden.
4. Increase the heat to high and put in the chicken. Cook while stirring continuously, for roughly one minute.
5. Put in the green onions and onion slices and cook for half a minute.
6. Put in the Chili Tamarind Paste, broth, oyster sauce, fish sauce, and sugar. Continue to stir-fry for 30 more seconds.
7. Put in the reserved chilies and the cashews; stir-fry for 1 more minute or until the chicken is thoroughly cooked and the onions are soft.

Yield: Servings 2–4

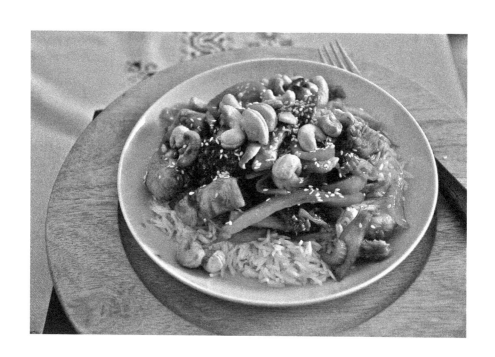

THAI GLAZED CHICKEN

Ingredients:

- 1 tablespoon fish sauce
- 1 tablespoon minced cilantro
- 1 teaspoon chopped ginger
- 1 teaspoon salt
- 1 teaspoon white pepper
- 1 whole chicken, cut in half (ask your butcher to do this for you)
- 2 tablespoons coconut milk
- 2 tablespoons rice wine
- 2 tablespoons soy sauce
- 4 cloves garlic, chopped

Directions:

1. Wash the chicken under cold water, then pat dry. Trim off any surplus fat or skin. Put the chicken halves in big Ziplock bags.
2. Mix the rest of the ingredients together in a small container until well blended.

3. Pour the marinade into the Ziplock bags, seal closed, and turn until the chicken is uniformly coated with the marinade. Allow the chicken to marinate for thirty minutes to an hour in your fridge.
4. Preheat your oven to 350 degrees.
5. Take away the chicken from the bags and put them breast side up in a roasting pan big enough to hold them easily. (Discard the rest of the marinade.)
6. Roast the chicken for about forty-five minutes.
7. Turn on the broiler and broil for roughly ten minutes or until done.

Yield: Servings 2–4

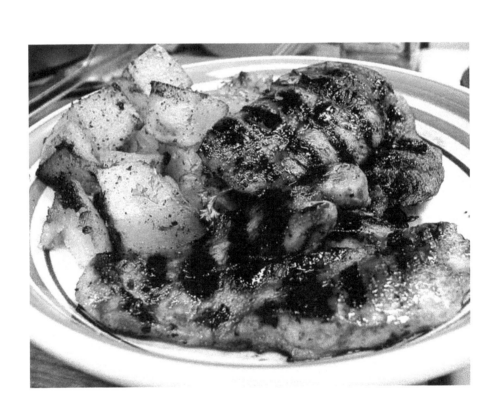

THAI-STYLE GREEN CURRY CHICKEN

Ingredients:

- ¼ cup (or to taste) chopped cilantro leaves ¼ cup Green Curry Paste ¼ cup vegetable oil
- 2 cups coconut milk
- 3 tablespoons fish sauce
- 3 whole boneless, skinless chicken breasts, cut into bite-sized pieces
- Steamed white rice

Directions:

1. Heat 2 tablespoons of vegetable oil in a big sauté pan or wok on moderate heat. Put in the chicken and sauté until mildly browned on all sizes. Take away the chicken and save for later.
2. Put in the remaining vegetable oil to the sauté pan. Mix in the curry paste and cook for two to three minutes. Put in the coconut milk and carry on cooking for five minutes. Put in the reserved chicken and fish sauce. Decrease the heat and simmer until chicken is soft, fifteen to twenty minutes. Mix in the cilantro.
3. Serve with steamed white rice.

Yield: Servings 4–6

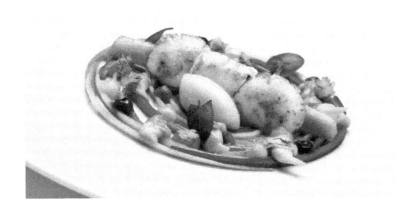

BASIL SCALLOPS

Ingredients:

- ¼ cup shredded bamboo shoots
- ½ pound bay scallops, cleaned
- 1 (14-ounce) can straw mushrooms, drained
- 2 tablespoons vegetable oil
- 3 cloves garlic, chopped
- 3 kaffir lime leaves, julienned, or the peel of 1 small lime cut into fine strips
- 3 tablespoons oyster sauce
- fifteen–20 fresh basil leaves

Directions:

1. In a wok or frying pan, heat the oil on high. Put in the garlic and lime leaves, and stir-fry until aromatic, approximately fifteen seconds.
2. Put in the scallops, mushrooms, bamboo shoots, and oyster sauce; continue to stir-fry for roughly four to five minutes or until the scallops are done to your preference.
3. Stir in the basil leaves and serve instantly.

Yield: Servings 2–4

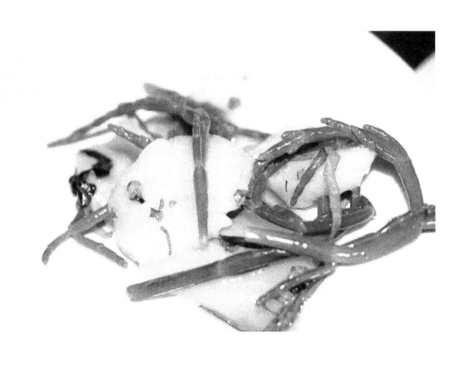

BROILED SALMON WITH 5-SPICE LIME BUTTER

Ingredients:

- ¼–½ teaspoon Chinese 5-spice powder
- 1 tablespoon unsalted butter
- 2 (6-ounce) salmon fillets, washed and patted dry
- 2 teaspoons lime juice
- Vegetable oil

Directions:

1. Using paper towels, wipe a thin coat of vegetable oil over a broiler pan.
2. Preheat your broiler on high, with the rack set on the upper third of the oven.
3. Melt the butter using low heat in a small deep cooking pan. Mix in the 5-spice powder and lime juice; keep warm.
4. Put the salmon on the broiler pan, skin side up. Broil for two to 4 minutes or until the skin is crunchy. Turn the salmon over and broil two minutes more or until done to your preference.
5. Move the salmon to 2 plates and spoon the butter sauce over the top.

Yield: Servings 2

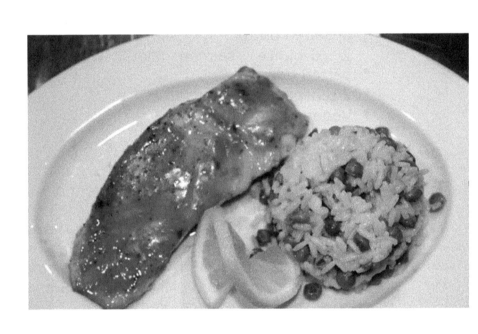

CLAMS WITH HOT BASIL

Ingredients:

- 1 bunch basil (Thai variety preferred), trimmed and julienned
- 1 tablespoon vegetable oil
- 2 cloves garlic
- 2 pounds Manila clams, cleaned
- 2 small dried red chili peppers, crushed
- 2 teaspoons sugar
- 4 teaspoons fish sauce

Directions:

1. Heat the oil in a big frying pan on high. Put in the chili peppers, garlic, and clams. Mix the clams until they open, approximately 4 to five minutes. Discard any clams that stay closed.
2. Put in the fish sauce and sugar; stir until well blended.
3. Put in the basil and stir until it wilts.
4. Serve instantly either as an appetizer or with rice as a main course.

Yield: Servings 4–6

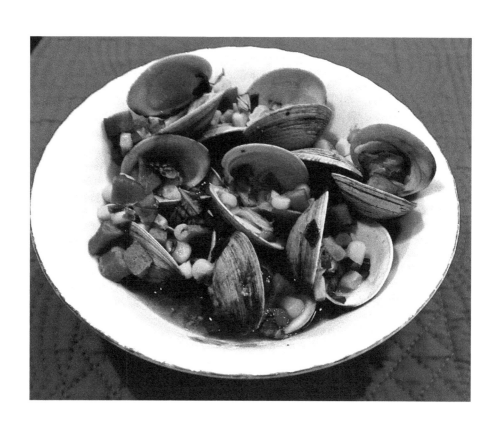

CURRIED MUSSELS

Ingredients:

- ½ cup sour cream
- ½ cup sweet white wine, such as Riesling 1 tablespoon lemon juice
- 1 teaspoon (or to taste) curry powder
- 2 pounds mussels, debearded and washed well
- 2 shallots, minced
- 2 tablespoons butter

Directions:

1. In a pan big enough to hold all of the mussels, melt the butter on moderate heat. Put in the shallots and sauté until tender and translucent.
2. Put in the wine and the mussels and raise the heat to high. Cover and cook, shaking the pan once in a while, until the mussels open, roughly ten minutes.
3. Take away the mussels from the pan, discarding any mussels that haven't opened.

Strain the pan liquid through a strainer and return it to the pan. Bring to its boiling point, then mix in the sour cream and curry powder.

4. Lower the heat to moderate-low and put in the lemon juice. Cook for two to three minutes. Tweak the seasonings of the sauce if required with salt and curry powder.
5. Return the mussels to the broth, coating them. Reheat before you serve.

Yield: Servings 2–4

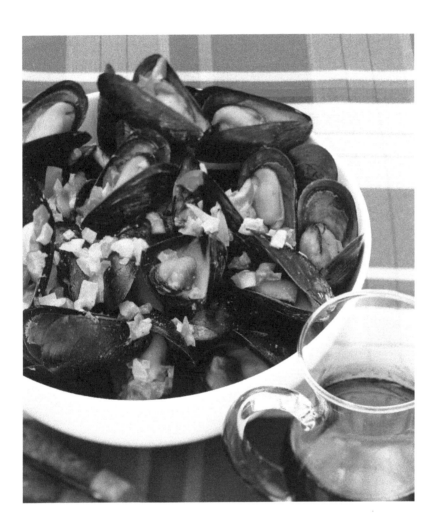

CURRIED SHRIMP WITH PEAS

Ingredients:

- 1 (10-ounce) package thawed frozen peas
- 1 (14-ounce) can unsweetened coconut milk
- 1 cup packed basil leaves, chopped
- 1 cup packed cilantro, chopped
- 1 tablespoon vegetable oil
- 1½ teaspoons <u>Red Curry Paste</u> (Page 17)
  2 pounds big shrimp, peeled and deveined
- 2–3 teaspoons brown
- sugar
- 4 teaspoons fish sauce
  Jasmine rice, cooked in accordance with
- package directions

Directions:

1. In a big pot, mix the curry paste, vegetable oil, and ¼ cup of the coconut milk; cook on moderate heat for one to two minutes.
2. Mix in the rest of the coconut milk and cook for an extra five minutes.
3. Put in the fish sauce and sugar, and cook for a minute more.
4. Put in the shrimp, basil, and cilantro; decrease the heat slightly and cook for four to five minutes or until the shrimp are almost done.
5. Put in the peas and cook two minutes more.
6. Serve over Jasmine rice.

Yield: Servings 4–6

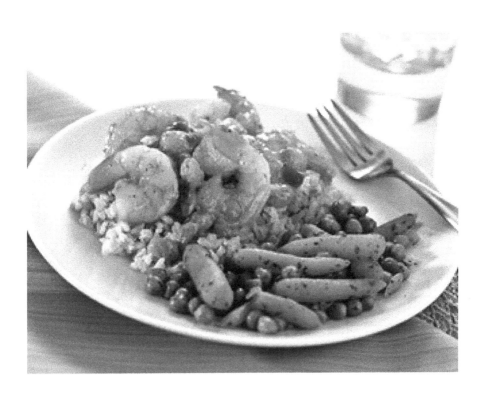

LIME-GINGER FILLETS

Ingredients:

- ½ teaspoon ground ginger
- ½ teaspoon salt
- 2 teaspoons lime zest
- 4 fish fillets, such as whitefish, perch, or pike
- 4 tablespoons unsalted butter, at room temperature Salt and
- freshly ground black pepper

Directions:

1. Preheat your broiler.
2. In a small container, meticulously mix the butter, lime zest, ginger, and ½ teaspoon salt.
3. Lightly flavor the fillets with salt and pepper and place on a baking sheet.
4. Broil for about four minutes. Brush each fillet with some of the lime-ginger butter and continue to broil for a minute or until the fish is done to your preference.

Yield: Servings 2–4

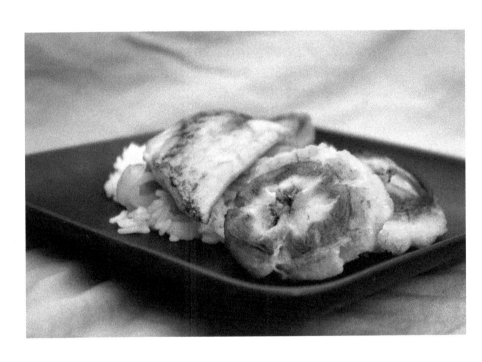

MARINATED STEAMED FISH

Ingredients:

- 1 big mushroom, thinly cut
- 1 tablespoon cut jalapeño pepper
- 1 tablespoon shrimp paste
- 1 tablespoon soy sauce
- 1 teaspoon Tabasco
- 1 whole lean flatfish (such as redfish, flounder, or bass), cleaned
- 2 green onions, finely cut
- 2 tablespoons grated ginger
- 3 tablespoons fish sauce
- Vegetable oil

Directions:

1. Swiftly wash the fish under cold water. Pat dry using paper towels. Using a sharp knife, deeply score the fish three to 4 times on each side.
2. Mix together all of the rest of the ingredients except the vegetable oil.
3. Put the fish in a big plastic bag. Pour the marinade over the fish and seal. Allow the fish to marinate for approximately 1 hour in your fridge.
4. Fill the base of a tiered steamer full of water. Bring the water to its boiling point.
5. Meanwhile, lightly coat the rack with vegetable oil. Put the fish on the rack.
6. Put the rack over the boiling water, cover, and allow to steam for fifteen to twenty minutes, until the flesh of the fish appears opaque when pierced using a knife.

Yield: Servings 4

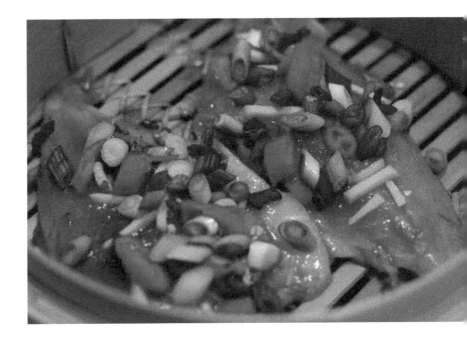

QUICK ASIAN-GRILLED FISH

Ingredients:

- 1 tablespoon cut jalapeño chili peppers
- 1 teaspoon freshly ground black pepper
- 1 whole fish, such as sea bass or mackerel, cleaned
- 2 teaspoons brown sugar
- 3 tablespoons chopped garlic, divided
- 3 tablespoons lime juice
- 4 tablespoons chopped cilantro

Directions:

1. Swiftly wash the fish under cold water. Pat dry using paper towels. Set the fish on a big sheet of aluminium foil.
2. Put the cilantro, 2 tablespoons of the garlic, and the black pepper in a food processor and process to make a thick paste.
3. Rub the paste all over the fish, both inside and out. Firmly wrap the fish in the foil.
4. To make the sauce, place the rest of the garlic, the lime juice, jalapeño, and brown sugar in a food processor and pulse until blended.
5. Put the fish on a prepared grill and cook for five to six minutes per side or until the flesh appears opaque when pierced using the tip of a knife.
6. Serve the fish with the sauce.

Yield: Servings 4–6

ROASTED SOUTHEAST ASIAN FISH

Ingredients:

- ¼ cup chopped green onion
- 1 teaspoon salt
- 12 fresh cilantro sprigs
- 3 cloves garlic
- 4 (12-inch-square) pieces of aluminium foil
  4 (8-ounce) fish fillets (salmon or mackerel
- are good choices)
  4 small fresh red chilies, seeded, 2 left whole
- and 2 julienned
- 4 thin slices of gingerroot
- 8 thin lime slices, cut in half
- Zest of 1 lime

Directions:

1. Use a food processor to mix the green onions, garlic, gingerroot, the 2 seeded whole chilies, the lime zest, and salt.
2. Preheat your oven to 450 degrees.
3. Wash the fish under cold water and pat dry. Put each fillet in the middle of a piece of foil. Rub liberally with the green onion paste. Top with the cilantro leaves, lime slices, and julienned chilies. Cover the fish in the foil.
4. Put the fish on a baking sheet and roast for roughly ten minutes per inch of thickness.
5. To serve, place unopened packets on each plate. Let guests unwrap.

Yield: Servings 4

SEAFOOD STIR-FRY

Ingredients:

- ¼ cup chopped basil
- 1 can bamboo shoots, washed and drained
- 1 pound fresh shrimp, scallops, or other seafood, cleaned
- 1 stalk lemongrass, bruised
- 2 shallots, chopped
- 3 tablespoons fish sauce
- 3 tablespoons vegetable oil
- 3 teaspoons garlic, chopped
- Pinch of brown sugar
- Rice, cooked in accordance with package directions

Directions:

1. Heat the oil in a frying pan or wok using high heat. Put in the garlic, shallots, lemongrass, and basil, and sauté for one to two minutes.
2. Decrease the heat, put in the rest of the ingredients, and stir-fry until the seafood is done to your preference, roughly five minutes.
3. Serve over rice.

Yield: Servings 2–4

SEARED COCONUT SCALLOPS

Ingredients:

- ¼ teaspoon cayenne
- ½ teaspoon salt
- 1 big egg, beaten
- 10 medium sea scallops, cleaned, washed, and patted dry 1½ cups
- sweetened, flaked coconut
- 2 cups boiling water
- Salt and pepper

Directions:

1. Preheat your oven to 350 degrees.
2. Put the coconut in a small container. Pour the boiling water over the coconut, stir, and then drain through a colander. Pat dry.
3. Spread the coconut on a baking sheet and bake for about ten minutes or until golden.
4. Put the toasted coconut in a small container and mix in the cayenne and salt.
5. Flavour the scallops with salt and pepper.
6. Heat a heavy, nonstick pan using high heat until almost smoking.
7. Immerse each scallop in the beaten egg, letting most of the egg drip off, then press the scallops into the coconut mixture.
8. Put the scallops in the pan and sear for one to 1½ minutes per side until just done.

Yield: Servings 2

SNAPPER BAKED WITH FISH SAUCE AND GARLIC

Ingredients:

- ¼ cup fish sauce
- 1 tablespoon sesame oil
- 2 cloves garlic, minced
- 2 whole small red snappers, cleaned but left whole

Directions:

1. Using a sharp knife, make 3 deep diagonal slits on each side of the fish. Put the fish in an ovenproof baking dish.
2. Mix the fish sauce, sesame oil, and garlic in a small container. Ladle the mixture over the fish, ensuring it goes into the slits. Allow the fish to sit at room temperature for half an hour
3. Bake the fish in a 425-degree oven for thirty minutes or until the skin is crunchy.

Yield: Servings 2

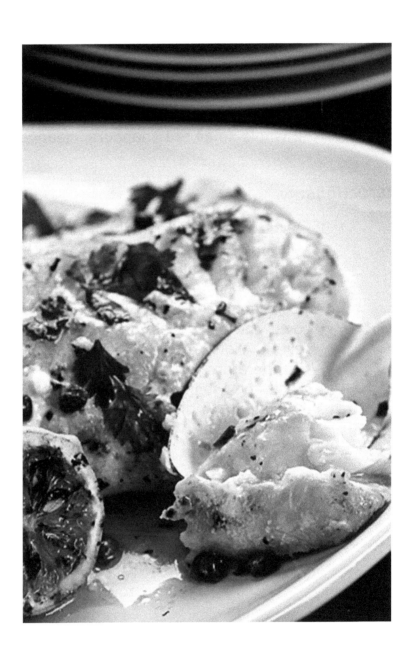

STEAMED MUSSELS WITH LEMONGRASS

Ingredients:

- 1 serrano chili
- 2 pounds mussels, cleaned
- 2 stalks lemongrass, outer leaves removed and discarded, inner portion bruised
- 3 (½-inch) slices unpeeled ginger
- 3 cups water
- 5 cloves garlic
- Peel of 1 lime
- Tabasco to taste

Directions:

1. Put the water, lemongrass, lime, garlic, and ginger in a pot big enough to hold all of the mussels. Bring to its boiling point, reduce heat, and allow to simmer for five minutes.
2. Bring the liquid back to its boiling point and put in the mussels; cover and allow to steam for five minutes, shaking the pan every so frequently.
3. Move the mussels to a serving platter, discarding any mussels that have not opened.
4. Put in the chili pepper to the broth and simmer for another two minutes. Strain the broth, then pour over the mussels.
5. Serve the mussels with Tabasco on the side.

Yield: Servings 2–4

STEAMED RED SNAPPER

Ingredients:

- 1 recipe Thai Sauce of your choice
- 1 whole red snapper (about 2 pounds), cleaned, but left whole Vegetable oil

Directions:

1. Swiftly wash the fish under cold water. Pat dry using paper towels. Using a sharp knife, deeply score the fish three to 4 times on each side.
2. Fill the base of a tiered steamer full of water. Bring the water to its boiling point.
3. Meanwhile, lightly coat the steamer rack with vegetable oil. Put the fish on the rack.
4. Put the rack over the boiling water, cover, and allow to steam for ten to twelve minutes, until the flesh of the fish appears opaque when pierced using a knife.
5. Serve the sauce on the side.

Yield: Servings 4

STIR-FRIED SHRIMP AND GREEN BEANS

Ingredients:

- ½ cup cleaned shrimp
- 1 tablespoon <u>Red Curry Paste</u> (Page 17)
- 1 tablespoon vegetable oil
- 1½ cups green beans, trimmed and slice into 1-inch lengths 2 teaspoons fish sauce
- 2 teaspoons sugar

Directions:

1. Heat the vegetable oil on moderate heat. Mix in the curry paste and cook for a minute to release the fragrance.
2. Put in the shrimp and the green beans at the same time, and stir-fry until the shrimp become opaque. (The green beans will still be fairly crunchy. If you prefer your beans softer, cook an additional minute.)
3. Put in the fish sauce and the sugar; stir until blended.
4. Serve instantly with rice.

Yield: Servings 2–3

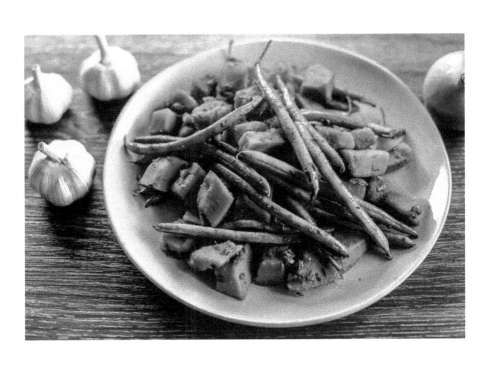

ASIAN GRILLED VEGETABLES

Ingredients:

- 1 recipe Asian Marinade
- 1 summer squash, cut into 1-inch slices
- 1 zucchini, cut into 1-inch slices
- 12 whole mushrooms, roughly 1-inch in diameter
- 12 whole pearl onions or 12 (2-inch) pieces of white onion 2 bell peppers
- (red, yellow, or green, in any combination), seeded and slice into two-inch squares

Directions:

1. Alternate the vegetables on 6 skewers (soak the skewers in water until tender if using wooden skewers).
2. Put the skewers in a pan big enough to let them lay flat. Pour the marinade over the skewers and allow it to sit for roughly 1 hour.
3. Put the skewers in a mildly oiled grill basket and place on a hot grill. Cook roughly five minutes on each side or until vegetables are done to your preference.

Yield: Servings 6

CURRIED GREEN BEANS

Ingredients:

- 1 pound green beans, trimmed Steamed rice
- 2 tablespoons Red Curry Paste (Page 17)
- 2 tablespoons vegetable oil
- 6 cups chicken or vegetable both

Directions:

1. In a big deep cooking pan, heat the vegetable oil on moderate to high heat.
2. Put in the curry paste and stir-fry for a minute.
3. Mix in the broth until well blended with the paste. Put in the green beans and bring to a low boil. Cook for fifteen to twenty minutes to reduce the liquid.
4. Lower the heat to sustain a hard simmer and carry on cooking until the beans are very well done.
5. Serve the beans over steamed rice, ladling the sauce over the top.

Yield: Servings 4–6

GINGERED GREEN BEANS

Ingredients:

- ¼ teaspoon salt
- ½ cup coconut milk
- ½ pound green beans, trimmed
- 1 stalk lemongrass, minced (inner soft portion only)
- 1 tablespoon peeled and minced ginger
- 1–3 (to taste) serrano chilies, seeded and minced 2
- tablespoons vegetable oil

Directions:

1. In a moderate-sized-sized deep cooking pan, heat the oil on moderate to high. Mix in the lemongrass, ginger, and chilies; sauté for one to two minutes.
2. Mix in the coconut milk and the salt until well blended.
3. Put in the green beans, raise the heat to high, and cook for about three minutes or until the beans are done to your preference.

Yield: Servings 2–4

GREEN BEANS WITH MACADAMIA NUT SAUCE

Ingredients:

- ½ teaspoon cayenne pepper
- ½ teaspoon ground cumin
- ½-1 teaspoon salt to taste
- 1 bay leaf
- 1 cup coconut milk
- 1 medium onion, chopped
- 1 pound green beans, trimmed
- 1 teaspoon ground coriander
- 2 cloves garlic, chopped
- 2 tablespoons vegetable oil
- 2 tablespoons water
- 4 whole raw macadamia nuts, chopped

Directions:

1. Put the onion, macadamia nuts, garlic, vegetable oil, and water in a blender or food processor and process until the desired smoothness is achieved. Move the paste to a small container and mix in the cayenne pepper, coriander, and cumin.
2. In a moderate-sized-sized deep cooking pan, heat the macadamia nut paste, coconut milk, and bay leaf on moderate to high heat. Heat to a simmer, reduce heat, and cook until reduced to half.
3. Mix in the salt. Put in the green beans and continue simmering, stirring once in a while, until the beans are done to your preference, approximately eight to ten minutes. Put in salt to taste if required.

Yield: Servings 4–6

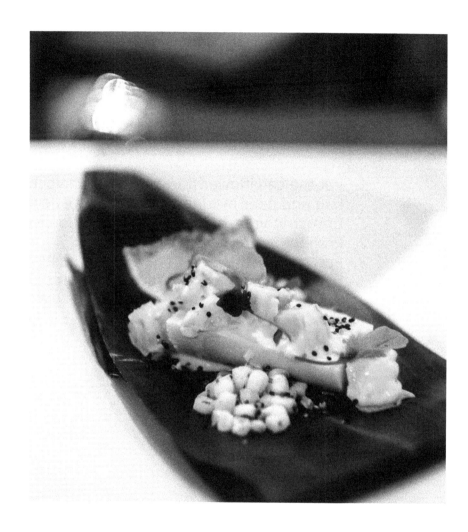

ROASTED ASIAN CAULIFLOWER

Ingredients:

- 1 head cauliflower, broken into florets (cut the florets in half if large)

Directions:

1. Put the cauliflower florets in a big Ziplock bag and pour marinade over them; allow to rest in your fridge for four to 6 hours.
2. Preheat your oven to 500 degrees.
3. Put the cauliflower florets in a roasting pan. Roast for roughly fifteen minutes or until soft, turning after seven to eight minutes.

Yield: Servings 6–8

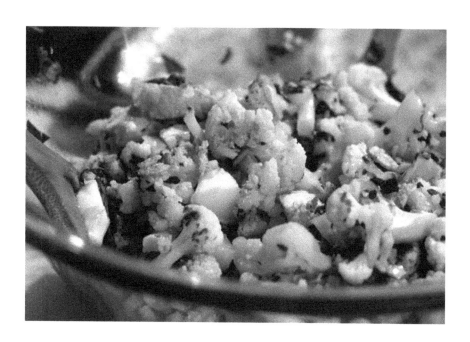

GRILLED EGGPLANT WITH AN ASIAN TWIST

Ingredients:

- 4—8 Japanese eggplants (approximately 1½ pounds in all)
- Olive oil
- Salt and pepper to taste

Directions:

1. Prepare a grill or broiler. Let it achieve high heat.
2. If the eggplants are relatively large, cut in half vertically. Toss them with a little olive oil just to coat, and sprinkle with salt and pepper. Put the eggplant either in a vegetable grilling basket or directly on the grill grate or broiler pan. Cook until soft, approximately fifteen to twenty minutes, turning midway through the cooking process.
3. Turn off the heat. Drizzle with lemon juice and fish sauce.
4. Decorate using basil leaves. Serve either hot or at room temperature.

Yield: Servings 4–6

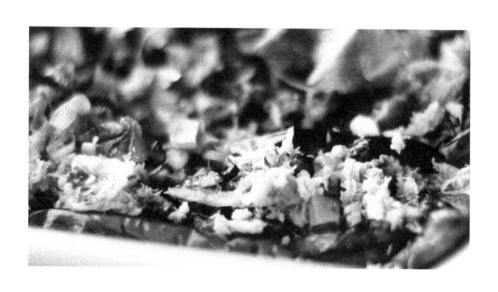

JAPANESE EGGPLANT WITH TOFU

Ingredients:

- 3 cups cut Japanese eggplant, approximately -inch thick ¼ pound
- extra-firm tofu, cut into little cubes
- 2–3 cloves garlic, finely chopped
- 4–6 tablespoons vegetable oil

Directions:

1. Heat the oil in a big frying pan on moderate to high heat. Put in the garlic and sauté until it turns golden.
2. Put in the eggplant and tofu pieces; sauté, stirring continuously, for five to six minutes or until the eggplant is done to your preference.
3. Cautiously mix in the rest of the ingredients.
4. Serve instantly to avoid discoloration of the eggplant and basil.

Yield: Servings 2–4

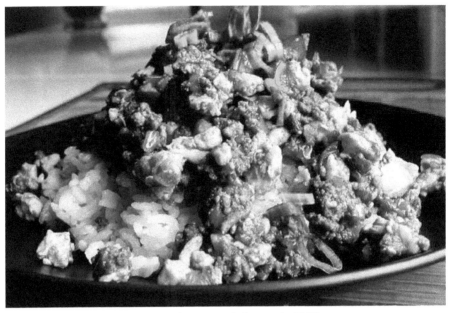

PUMPKIN WITH PEPPERCORNS AND GARLIC

Ingredients:

- 1 tablespoon vegetable oil
- 2 cloves garlic
  2 cups fresh pumpkin pieces, cut into 1-inch
- cubes
- 30 peppercorns

Directions:

1. Using a mortar and pestle, crush together the peppercorns and the garlic.
2. Put in the vegetable oil to a big sauté pan and heat on high. Put in the peppercorn-garlic mixture and stir-fry until the garlic just starts to brown.
3. Put in the pumpkin pieces, stirring to coat.
4. Put in the water and bring the water to a simmer. After the water has been reduced to half, mix in the fish sauce and sugar.
5. Continue to cook until the pumpkin is soft but not mushy.
6. Serve as a side dish.

Yield: Servings 4–6

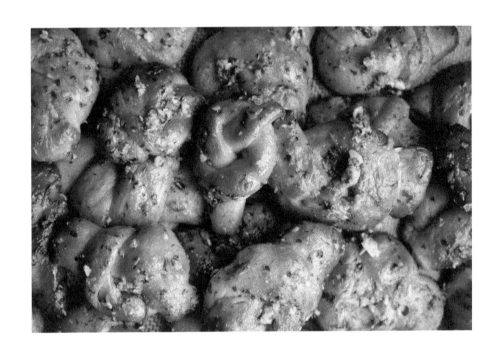

SOUTHEASTERN VEGETABLE STEW

Ingredients:

- ½ cup chopped cilantro
- 1 can straw mushrooms, drained
- 1 Chinese cabbage, cut into bite-sized pieces
- 1 cup cut leeks
- 1 tablespoon minced ginger
- 1 teaspoon vegetable oil
- 1 Western cabbage, quartered, cored, and slice into bitesized pieces
- 2 cups cut celery
- 2 tablespoons brown sugar
- 2 tablespoons dark soy sauce
- 3 cups bean noodles, soaked, and slice into short lengths
- 3 tablespoons chopped garlic
- 3 tablespoons fish sauce
- 4 cups roughly chopped kale
- 4 cups turnip, cut into bitesized pieces
- 5 cakes hard tofu, cut into bite-sized pieces
- 6 tablespoons soybean paste
- 8 cups vegetable stock
- Freshly ground pepper to taste

Directions:

1. Bring the stock to its boiling point and put in the fish sauce, soy sauce, brown sugar.
2. Reduce the heat, put in the vegetables and tofu, and simmer vegetables are nearly soft.
3. In a small sauté pan, heat the oil on moderate heat. Put in paste and stir-fry until aromatic. Put in the garlic and ginger, until the garlic is golden.
4. Put in the soybean paste mixture to the soup. Mix in the noodles and cilantro, and simmer 5 more minutes.
5. Flavor it with the pepper and additional fish sauce to taste.

Yield: Servings 8

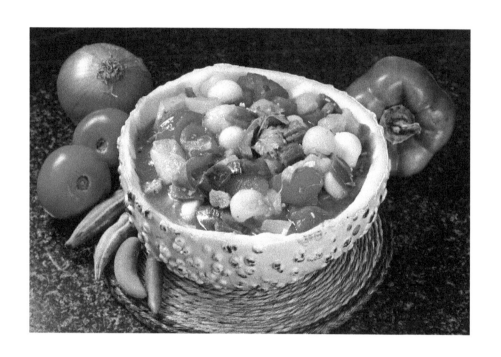

SPICY STIR-FRIED CORN

Ingredients:

- 1 cup low-sodium vegetable broth
- 1 medium onion, minced
- 1 stalk lemongrass, minced (soft inner portion only)
- 1 tablespoon butter
- 2 tablespoons fish sauce Tabasco to taste
- 2 tablespoons lime juice
- 2 tablespoons vegetable oil
- 2 teaspoons lime zest
- 2 teaspoons minced garlic
- 4 cups corn kernels (fresh or frozen and thawed are best)

Directions:

1. Put the oil in a big frying pan using high heat. Put in the lemongrass. Once it starts to brown, put in the garlic, butter, and onion. Continue to cook on high, letting the ingredients brown fairly.
2. Put in the corn kernels and cook until they brown. Mix in the vegetable stock; stirring continuously, cook the mixture for a couple of minutes, scraping the bottom of the pan to loosen any burned-on bits.
3. Mix in the rest of the ingredients and cook for 30 more seconds.

Yield: Servings 6–8

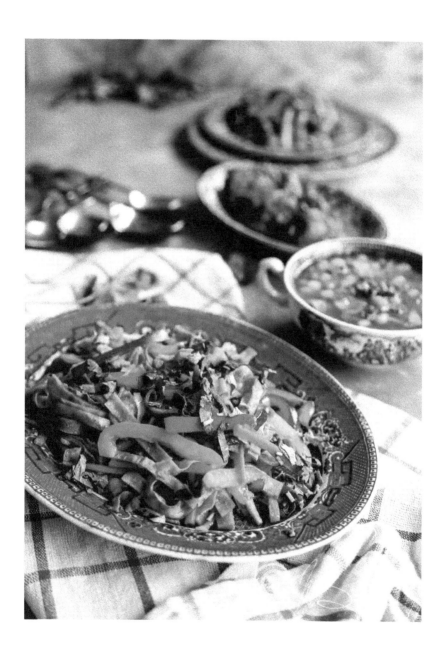

STIR-FRIED BLACK MUSHROOMS AND ASPARAGUS

Ingredients:

- 1 ounce dried Chinese black mushrooms
- 1 pound asparagus spears, trimmed
- 1 tablespoon vegetable oil
- 1-2 cloves garlic, minced

Directions:

1. Put the dried mushrooms in a container and cover with hot water. Allow to soak for fifteen minutes. Drain, discard the stems, and slice into strips; set aside.
2. Heat the oil on moderate to high in a big frying pan. Put in the garlic and sauté until golden.
3. Mix in the mushrooms and carry on cooking, stirring continuously, for a minute.
4. Mix in the oyster sauce and a few drops of Tabasco if you wish.
5. Put in the asparagus spears. Sauté for two to 4 minutes or until the asparagus is done to your preference.

Yield: Servings 4-6

THAI PICKLED VEGETABLES

Ingredients:

- ½ cup bok choy
- ½ cup cilantro leaves
- 1 big cucumber, seeded and slice into 3-inch-long, ½-inch wide strips
- 1 cup baby corn
- 1 cup broccoli florets
- 1 cup cut carrots
- 1 recipe Thai Vinegar Marinade
- 2–3 tablespoons toasted sesame seeds 4 cups
- water

Directions:

1. Bring the water to its boiling point in a big pan. Put in the vegetables blanch for two to three minutes. Strain the vegetables and shock water to stop the cooking process.
2. Put the vegetables in a big container and pour the Thai Vinegar Marinade over the top. Allow to cool to room temperature and then place in your fridge for minimum 4 hours or maximum 2 weeks (yes, weeks).
3. Mix in the cilantro and sesame seeds just before you serve.

Yield: Approximately 6 cups

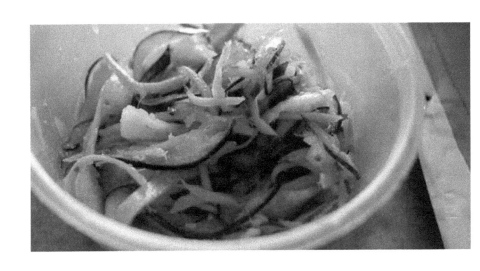

THAI VEGETABLE CURRY

Ingredients:

- ¼ cup Green Curry
- ½ cup fresh minced cilantro
- 1 pound Japanese eggplant, cut into 1-inch slices
- 1 pound small boiling potatoes, quartered (or halved if large)
- 12 ounces baby carrots
- 2 cups broccoli florets
- 2 tablespoons vegetable oil
- 3 cups canned, unsweetened coconut milk
- 3 tablespoons fish sauce
- 3—4 ounces green beans, cut into 1-inch lengths

Directions:

1. In a heavy stew pot, heat the oil. Put in the curry paste two to three minutes.
2. Put in the coconut milk and fish sauce; simmer for five minutes.
3. Put in the potatoes, eggplant, and carrots, and bring to a heat and simmer for about ten minutes. Put in the broccoli and carry on simmering until the vegetables are thoroughly cooked, ten minutes.
4. Just before you serve mix in the cilantro.

Yield: Servings 4–6

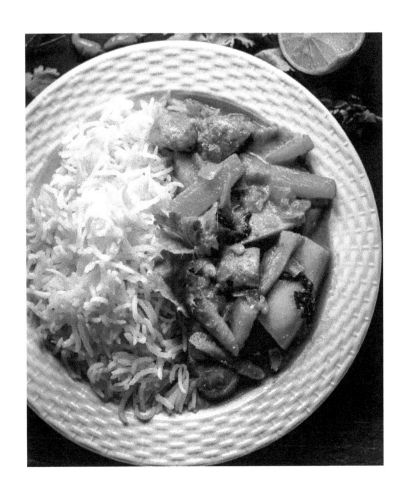

Lightning Source UK Ltd.
Milton Keynes UK
UKHW021333290421
382828UK00005B/44